About the NCCN Guidelines for Patients®

National Comprehensive Cancer Network®

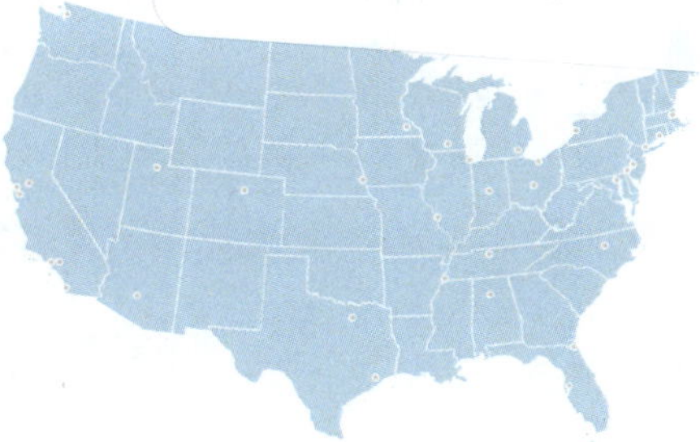

Did you know that top cancer centers across the United States work together to improve cancer care? This alliance of leading cancer centers is called the National Comprehensive Cancer Network® (NCCN®).

Cancer care is always changing. NCCN develops evidence-based cancer care recommendations used by health care providers worldwide. These frequently updated recommendations are the NCCN Clinical Practice Guidelines in Oncology (NCCN Guidelines®). The NCCN Guidelines for Patients plainly explain these expert recommendations for people with cancer and caregivers.

These NCCN Guidelines for Patients are based on the NCCN Clinical Practice Guidelines in Oncology (NCCN Guidelines®) for Gastrointestinal Stromal Tumors, Version 1.2023 – March 13, 2023.

View the NCCN Guidelines for Patients free online
NCCN.org/patientguidelines

Find an NCCN Cancer Center near you
NCCN.org/cancercenters

Connect with us

Supporters

NCCN Guidelines for Patients are supported by funding from the NCCN Foundation®

NCCN Foundation gratefully acknowledges the following corporate supporters for helping to make available these NCCN Guidelines for Patients: Boehringer Ingelheim Pharmaceuticals, Inc.; Deciphera, and SpringWorks Therapeutics, Inc.

NCCN independently adapts, updates and hosts the NCCN Guidelines for Patients. Our corporate supporters do not participate in the development of the NCCN Guidelines for Patients and are not responsible for the content and recommendations contained therein.

Additional support is provided by

Dottie Shead

To make a gift or learn more visit online or email

NCCNFoundation.org/donate

PatientGuidelines@NCCN.org

Contents

NCCN Foundation seeks to support the millions of patients and their families affected by a cancer diagnosis by funding and distributing NCCN Guidelines for Patients. NCCN Foundation is also committed to advancing cancer treatment by funding the nation's promising doctors at the center of innovation in cancer research. For more details and the full library of patient and caregiver resources, visit NCCN.org/patients.

National Comprehensive Cancer Network (NCCN) and NCCN Foundation
3025 Chemical Road, Suite 100, Plymouth Meeting, PA 19462 USA

1

GIST basics

Gastrointestinal stromal tumors (GIST) are a type of soft tissue sarcoma. GIST occur most often in the wall of the stomach or small bowel. Together, you and your cancer care team will decide on a treatment plan.

Overview

While all GIST are considered to be cancerous, their behavior can vary widely from person to person. Some GIST are small, slow-growing, and unlikely to spread. Others may be large and grow quickly, regrow after treatment, and spread to the liver or within the abdominal cavity.

Where GIST form

GIST can form anywhere within the walls of gastrointestinal (GI) tract. But they are most often found in the stomach, followed by the small intestine (also called the small bowel). Less commonly, GIST form in the rectum, colon, or esophagus. GIST that form outside the stomach tend to be more aggressive, but those within the stomach can also grow quickly.

Symptoms

A GIST can cause health changes you can feel or notice (symptoms). Other problems caused by a GIST can only be found by testing. Symptoms of GIST include:

- Feeling full quickly when eating
- Abdominal pain, swelling, or bloating
- Feeling sick to your stomach
- Blood in stool and/or blood in vomit
- Fatigue

Where GIST form

GIST are most often found in the stomach or small bowel but can occur anywhere in the GI tract.

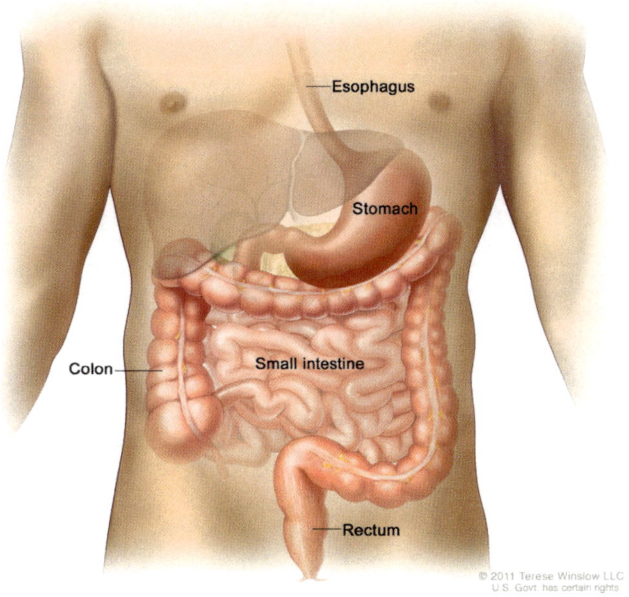

Testing

Imaging and a biopsy are needed to diagnose GIST, and to distinguish it from other types of tumors that occur in the GI tract. Your test results and treatment options should be reviewed by a team of experts with experience in treating this rare type of cancer.

Imaging

Abdomen and pelvis

If GIST is suspected, imaging of the abdomen and pelvis is needed. Expect to have computed tomography (CT) and/or magnetic resonance imaging (MRI).

A CT scan is a more detailed type of x-ray. It takes many images from different angles. A computer combines the images to make detailed pictures. During the scan, you will lie face up on a table that moves through a large doughnut-like machine. You will be alone during the scan, but a technician will be nearby. You will be able to hear and talk to them at all times. You may hear buzzing or clicking during the scan.

MRI uses strong magnetic fields and radio waves to make pictures of areas inside the body. It is especially good at making clear pictures of areas of soft tissue and the liver. Unlike a CT scan or x-ray, MRI does not use radiation. Those with certain types of heart monitors, pacemakers, or metal implants may not be able to have MRI. Talk to your doctor. Also, tell your care team if you get nervous in tight spaces. You may be given a medicine to help you relax.

During these scans, you may be given contrast. This substance helps make imaging pictures clearer. It may be injected into your vein or mixed with a liquid you drink. The contrast may cause you to feel warm or flushed. If you have an allergic reaction to contrast, you may develop a rash or have trouble breathing.

CT scan

A CT scan is a more detailed type of x-ray. It is painless and noninvasive. CT makes many images from different angles. A computer combines the images to make 3D pictures.

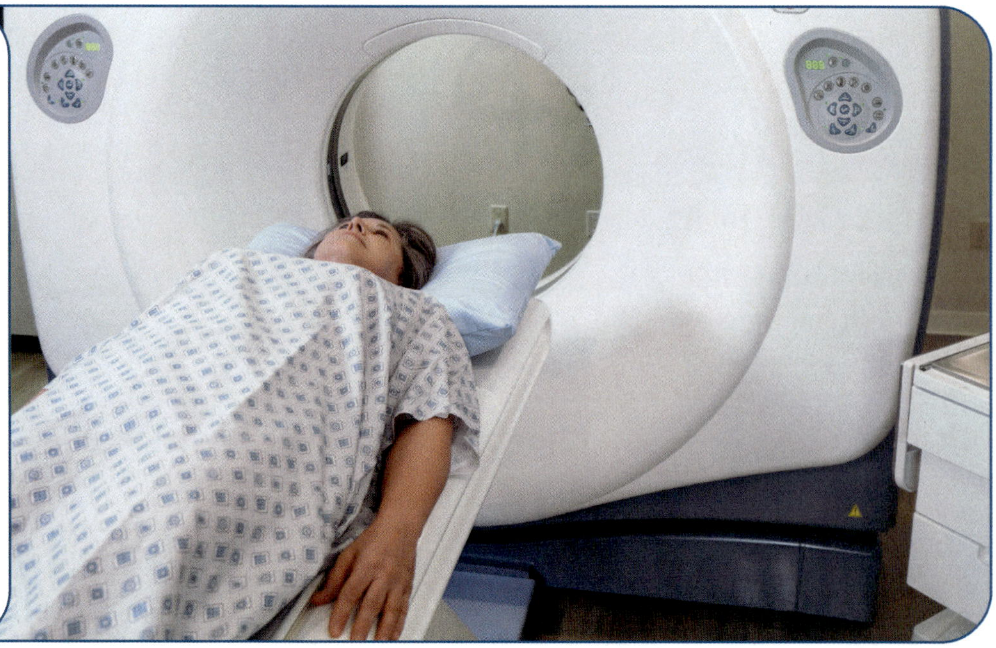

Chest

For a GIST that is 2 centimeters (about the size of a penny) or larger, imaging of the chest may also be recommended. The purpose is to look for signs of cancer spread. Either an x-ray or CT scan may be performed. X-rays are painless and use a small amount of radiation.

Biopsy

Your doctor may want to remove a small sample of the tumor for testing (a biopsy). If needed, an endoscopic ultrasound (EUS)-guided biopsy is recommended. A thin tube (endoscope) is inserted through the mouth. It is guided down the esophagus into the stomach. The endoscope has an ultrasound probe and a needle for removing a sample of the GIST. The ultrasound probe sends images to a monitor. This allows your doctor to see where to position the biopsy needle.

If a thin, hollow needle is used, it is called an EUS fine-needle aspiration biopsy (EUS-FNAB). This type removes a small amount of fluid and tumor tissue. Use of a slightly larger needle to remove a circular-shaped piece of tissue is called an EUS core needle biopsy (EUS-CNB). A pathologist examines the removed tissue under a microscope to determine whether the tumor is a GIST.

Biomarker testing

Knowing whether the tumor has certain features, called biomarkers, can help guide your treatment. Biomarkers are often genetic changes (mutations). The presence (or lack) of specific mutations or other biomarkers can affect how the GIST responds to certain targeted therapies.

If treatment with drug therapy is planned, the biopsy sample will be used for biomarker testing. Testing for many genetic biomarkers at one time is called next-generation sequencing (NGS). NGS can find gene mutations for which targeted treatments may be available. The results help your treatment team choose the best drug therapy for your GIST.

Chest x-ray

For a GIST larger than 2 cm, imaging of the chest with either x-ray or CT may be recommended. A chest x-ray (shown here) is painless and uses a very small amount of radiation.

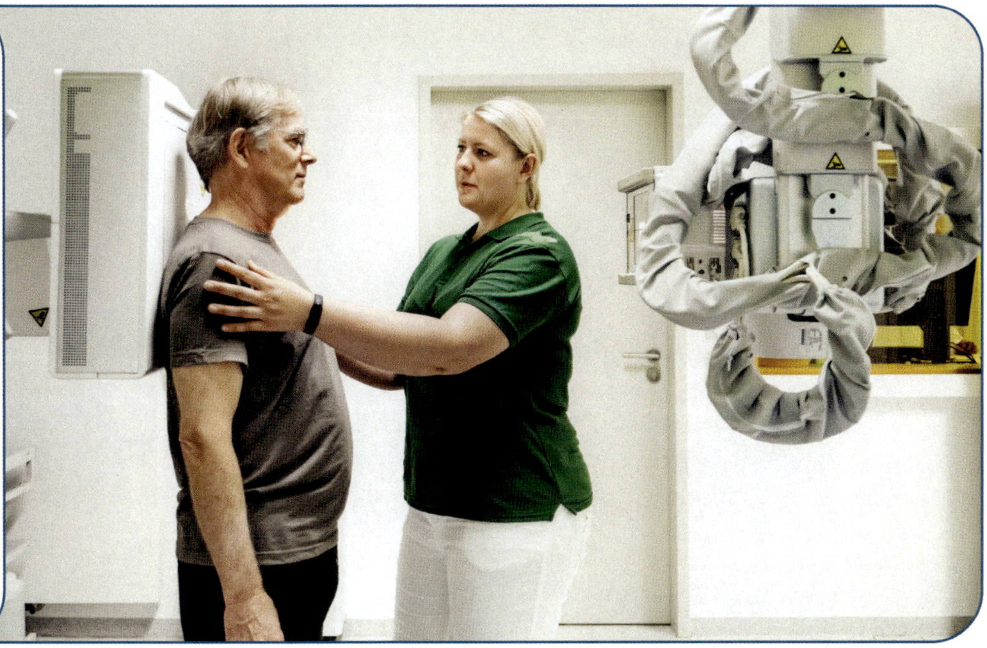

Other names for biomarker testing include molecular testing, tumor profiling, genomic testing, tumor gene testing, somatic genomic testing, and mutation testing.

KIT and *PDGFRA* gene mutations

Mutations in the *KIT* gene are the most common genetic changes found in GIST. About 7 to 8 out of 10 GIST have a *KIT* mutation. The next most common mutations are those in the platelet-derived growth factor receptor alpha (*PDGFRA*) gene. *PDGFRA* mutations are often found in stomach GIST.

KIT and *PDGFRA* mutations cause cells to grow. In most cases, *KIT* and *PDGFRA* mutations are acquired. This means they happen during a person's lifetime. If a GIST doesn't have either of these mutations, testing for *SDH* and other mutations (described next) is recommended.

SDH deficiency

For GIST without a *KIT* or *PDGFRA* mutation, testing to look for an *SDH* mutation is recommended. Succinate dehydrogenase (SDH) is a protein within cells that converts sugar to energy. Many GIST without a *KIT* or *PDGFRA* mutation have *SDH* deficiency. This means that a part of the *SDH* gene is inactive.

SDH-deficient GIST typically form in the stomach in younger people but can also be seen later in life. Four out of 5 grow slowly while others can be more aggressive. These are likely to spread in the body through lymph nodes, blood, or within the abdominal cavity. Referral to a genetic counselor for inherited (germline) testing is recommended for everyone with *SDH*-deficient GIST.

Other biomarkers

In addition to *SDH* deficiency, GIST without a *KIT* or *PDGFRA* mutation should be tested for other, rare biomarkers. These include *BRAF* mutations, *NF1* mutation, *NTRK* fusions, and *FGFR* fusions. Referral to a genetic counselor for inherited (germline) testing assessment is recommended for those with GIST that have *NF1* mutation.

GIST biomarkers

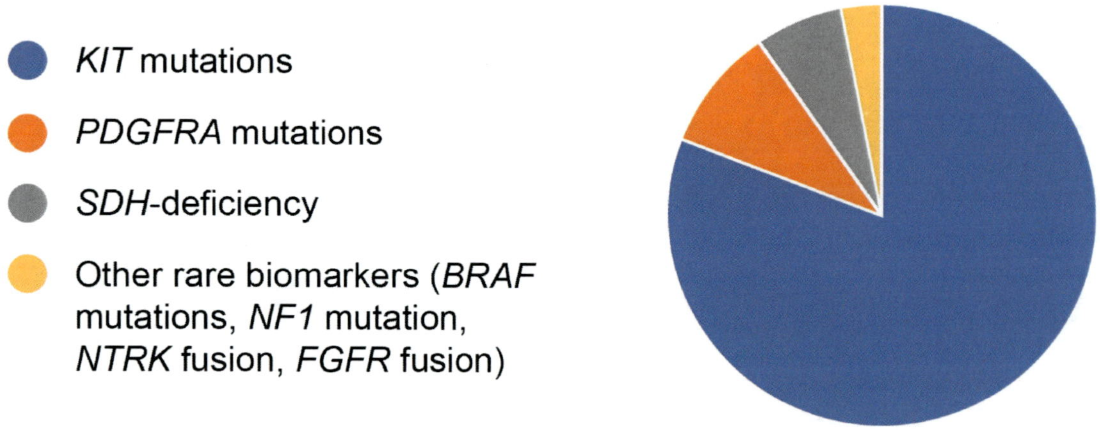

Staging

A combination of imaging and pathology (tumor tissue tests) are used to determine the stage of GIST.

The radiology report will include the size and location. The pathology report will include the size, location, and mitotic rate of the GIST. Mitotic rate is explained below. For GIST that have complex or unusual features, referral to a center that is experienced in sarcoma diagnosis is recommended.

The tumor, node, metastasis (TNM) staging system is used for GIST. The following factors are considered to determine the cancer stage.

Tumor size - The primary tumor is measured in centimeters (cm). For reference, a golf ball is 4 cm. A baseball is 7 cm. A grapefruit is 15 cm.

Spread to lymph nodes - Lymph nodes work as filters to help fight infection and remove harmful things from your body. Lymph nodes near the tumor are referred to as "regional." Spread to lymph nodes is rare for GIST, except in *SDH*-deficient, *NTRK*-fusion positive, or *FGFR*-fusion positive GIST. These tend to be less aggressive than other GIST.

Mitotic rate refers to how fast the cells make copies of themselves. A low mitotic rate is slower than a high mitotic rate. This can often only be determined after a tumor is removed, or if a sufficient amount of tissue is obtained at the time of biopsy.

Metastasis is the spread of cancer to distant areas. GIST most often spreads to the liver or to the lining of the abdomen (the peritoneum).

Stomach GIST

Stage I - GIST is smaller than 5 cm (stage IA) or between 5 and 10 cm (stage IB). The mitotic rate is low.

Stage II - The GIST may be small and have a high mitotic rate, or it may be large and have a low mitotic rate.

Stage III - The GIST is at least 5 cm and has a high mitotic rate.

Stage IV - The cancer has spread to nearby lymph nodes or to distant areas of the body (metastasized).

Small bowel GIST

Stage I – The GIST is smaller than 5 cm. The mitotic rate is low.

Stage II - The tumor is between 5 and 10 cm. The mitotic rate is low.

Stage IIIA - The tumor may be very small and have a high mitotic rate, or it may be large and have a low mitotic rate.

Stage IIIB - The tumor could be small or large. The mitotic rate is high.

Stage IV - The cancer has spread to nearby lymph nodes or to distant areas of the body (metastasized).

Key points

Overview

- Gastrointestinal stromal tumors (GIST) are fragile tumors that usually form in the stomach (most common) or small bowel.
- Test results and treatment options should be reviewed by a team of experts from different fields of surgery and medicine who have experience in treating GIST.

Testing

- Imaging of the abdomen and pelvis is needed for a suspected GIST. Expect to have CT, MRI, or both. Contrast should be used.
- For a GIST that is 2 cm or larger, a chest x-ray or chest CT may be recommended to look for cancer spread.
- If drug therapy is planned before surgery, a biopsy is needed to confirm GIST.
- If needed, the type of biopsy generally recommended for GIST is an endoscopic ultrasound (EUS)-guided needle biopsy.
- Biomarkers are features of a cancer that can help guide your treatment. Biomarkers are often genetic changes (mutations) in the tumor.
- The most common biomarkers in GIST are *KIT* gene mutations, followed by *PDGFRA* gene mutations.
- For a GIST without a *KIT* or *PDGFRA* mutation, testing to look for *SDH* deficiency and other rare biomarkers is recommended.

Staging

- The tumor, node, metastasis (TNM) staging system is used for GIST.
- The cancer is staged using tumor size, spread to lymph nodes, mitotic rate, and spread to distant areas (metastasis).

2

Treatment for GIST

Your test results and treatment options should be reviewed by a team of experts from different fields of surgery and medicine who have experience in treating gastrointestinal stromal tumors (GIST). This is called multidisciplinary cancer care.

Treatment

When possible, surgery is the recommended treatment for most GIST. If there is a high risk of complications from surgery, drug therapy may be given first. Some very small stomach GIST do not need treatment.

Very small stomach GIST

Stomach GIST smaller than 2 centimeters (cm) are unlikely to spread. Using the biopsy results (if performed) and imaging scans, your doctor will look for features that suggest the tumor will grow quickly. If high-risk features are found, an operation to remove the GIST is recommended. This is also called surgical resection. See "Treatment after surgery" on page 14 for next steps.

For very small stomach GIST without high-risk features, no treatment is needed. Instead, the tumor may be monitored with endoscopy or imaging tests. This option has risks. Talk with your doctor about whether surveillance is the best option for you.

All other GIST

Surgery to resect (remove) the GIST may be your first treatment. This is only possible if it does not put you at very high risk for complications. Depending on the size and location of the tumor, surgery can be difficult. GIST are fragile and easily rupture. In addition, nearby organs and tissues may be affected. Blood vessels might have to be removed, or pieces of them cut out and sewn back together. Parts of your stomach or other organs might have to be removed and reattached. Surgery to remove a GIST requires a great deal of skill.

The best possible surgical outcome is called complete resection or negative margin resection. Doctors call this "R0." This means that no tumor cells remain in the spot from which the tumor was removed (the "tumor bed"). All of the tumors must be removed in order to have a negative margin. This is not always possible.

If there is a high risk of serious problems from surgery, you may have drug therapy first. It can shrink the tumor and make surgery less risky. If drug therapy is planned, the tumor will be biopsied. This serves two main purposes. The biopsy sample is tested to confirm that the tumor is a GIST. The sample is also used for biomarker testing.

Biomarker testing is needed because some drug therapies work best in cancers with certain gene mutations or other biomarkers. For recommended drug therapy according to biomarker, see **Guide 1**. If the GIST does not have any of the biomarkers listed in **Guide 1**, drug therapy before surgery is <u>not</u> recommended. It is important to take your drug therapy, known as a tyrosine kinase inhibitor

(TKI), as directed. GIST may worsen if you stop taking your medicine or if you miss doses.

Before starting drug therapy, you will have a CT and/or MRI scan of your abdomen and pelvis. Your doctor might also order a PET/CT. During drug therapy, imaging will be used to check how treatment is working. Either a CT or MRI is recommended every 2 to 3 months. These results will be compared to your original (baseline) scans.

If the tumor **shrinks** or stops growing, drug therapy will be continued until your doctor feels it has provided all of the benefit it can. This may take 6 to 9 months, or more. At that time, your doctor and surgeon will decide if and when surgery is appropriate. After surgery, more treatment may be needed. See "Treatment after surgery." If the GIST **grows** during drug therapy and surgery does not become possible, see "Progression" on page 16.

It is hard to know the true extent of the cancer before surgery. The surgeon may find cancer in veins, arteries, or other organs. Ask your surgeon what might be removed during surgery and what this means in terms of healing and recovery time.

Guide 1
Drug therapy before surgery for high-risk candidates

Biomarker	Recommended drug therapy
***KIT* or *PDGFRA** mutations** ***except D842V and other *PDGFRA* mutations that don't respond to imatinib**	Imatinib (Gleevec)
***PDGFRA* mutations that don't respond to imatinib, including D842V**	Avapritinib (Ayvakit)
***SDH* deficiency**	Sunitinib (Sutent) or clinical trial (observation may also be considered)
***NTRK* fusions**	Larotrectinib (Vitrakvi) or entrectinib (Rozlytrek)
***BRAF* V600E mutation**	Dabrafenib (Tafinlar) + trametinib (Mekinist)

Treatment after surgery

If the results of surgery are very good, it is called "complete resection." In this case, you might start (or continue) taking imatinib. This depends on:

- the risk of recurrence based on features of the tumor, and
- whether you had drug therapy before surgery (and if so, the type)

If you were **not** on any type of drug therapy before surgery and the risk of recurrence is **low**, observation is recommended. Observation is also recommended for GIST without mutations that respond to imatinib.

If you were **not** on any type of drug therapy before surgery and the risk of recurrence is **high**, starting imatinib is recommended for GIST with mutations that respond to it.

If you were taking imatinib before surgery and the risk of recurrence is **high**, continuing imatinib is recommended.

If you were taking any of the drug therapies listed below before surgery, no further treatment is needed.

- Avapritinib (for some *PDGFRA* mutations)
- Larotrectinib (for *NTRK* fusions)
- Entrectinib (for *NTRK* fusions)
- Sunitinib (for *SDH*-deficiency)
- Dabrafenib + trametinib (for *BRAF* V600E mutation)

If you start (or continue) imatinib after surgery, talk to your doctor about how long you can expect to take it. There isn't a one-size-fits-all recommendation. The optimal length of drug therapy after surgery is unknown. For high-risk disease, it may be given for **at least** 3 years after surgery.

Surveillance after surgery

The return of cancer after treatment is called recurrence. Testing is used to find signs of recurrence early. This is called surveillance. Surveillance after **complete resection** of a GIST includes physical exams and imaging scans of your abdomen and pelvis.

These are recommended every 3 to 6 months for 5 years after surgery. For those at high risk of recurrence, testing every 3 months is recommended. After 5 years, most people have imaging and a physical exam once per year.

Some people may need less frequent surveillance. Those with low-risk or very small tumors may have imaging less often than described above. And those with high-risk tumors who stop TKI therapy may have imaging more often. Talk to your doctor about how often is right for you.

Tumor rupture

While rare, these fragile tumors may become damaged or punctured, causing cancer cells to spill into the abdomen. This can happen spontaneously or during surgery. If this happens, lifelong treatment with drug therapy is usually needed.

Recurrence or spread

Recurrent describes cancer that returns after treatment. Metastatic describes cancer that has spread to areas of the body far from where it started. Recurrent or metastatic GIST is treated with drug therapy. It is usually needed lifelong.

Imatinib is the preferred first-line therapy for GIST with mutations that respond to it, including most *PDGFRA* exon 18 mutations. Avapritinib is preferred for GIST with *PDGFRA* exon 18 mutations that do not respond to imatinib, including D842V.

If you are not a candidate for imatinib or avapritinib, you may have other options. This depends on the mutations found during biomarker testing. Options for less common biomarkers are listed below.

For *NTRK* gene fusion-positive GIST:
larotrectinib or entrectinib

For *SDH*-deficient GIST:
sunitinib, regorafenib, pazopanib, imatinib + binimetinib, or clinical trial

For *BRAF* V600E-mutated GIST:
dabrafenib + trametinib

Progression

The tumor may grow or spread while taking imatinib or avapritinib. If the new growth is limited, it may be possible to remove or control the cancer using local treatments. These include:

- Resection (surgery)
- Ablation, embolization, or chemoembolization (see next page for more information on these)
- Palliative radiation therapy to relieve symptoms

Another recommended option for progression is to switch to a different TKI. See the illustration below for the TKIs typically given after imatinib or avapritinib, and beyond.

An alternative recommended option may be increasing your imatinib dose, if you are taking standard-dose imatinib. This may work best in those with *KIT* exon 9 mutations.

If the new growth is widespread, switching TKIs or increasing the dose of imatinib is typically only considered for those who are fairly healthy otherwise. Doctors call this performance status. It is a rating of your ability to do daily tasks independently.

If GIST spreads or continues to grow despite treatment with the TKIs shown in the illustration, there are others that may be given. Your doctor may suggest doing another biopsy. The goal is to look for uncommon mutations that may have a corresponding targeted therapy. Consider enrolling in a clinical trial for treatment. Your care team can help you find

Systemic therapy for unresectable, progressive, or metastatic GIST

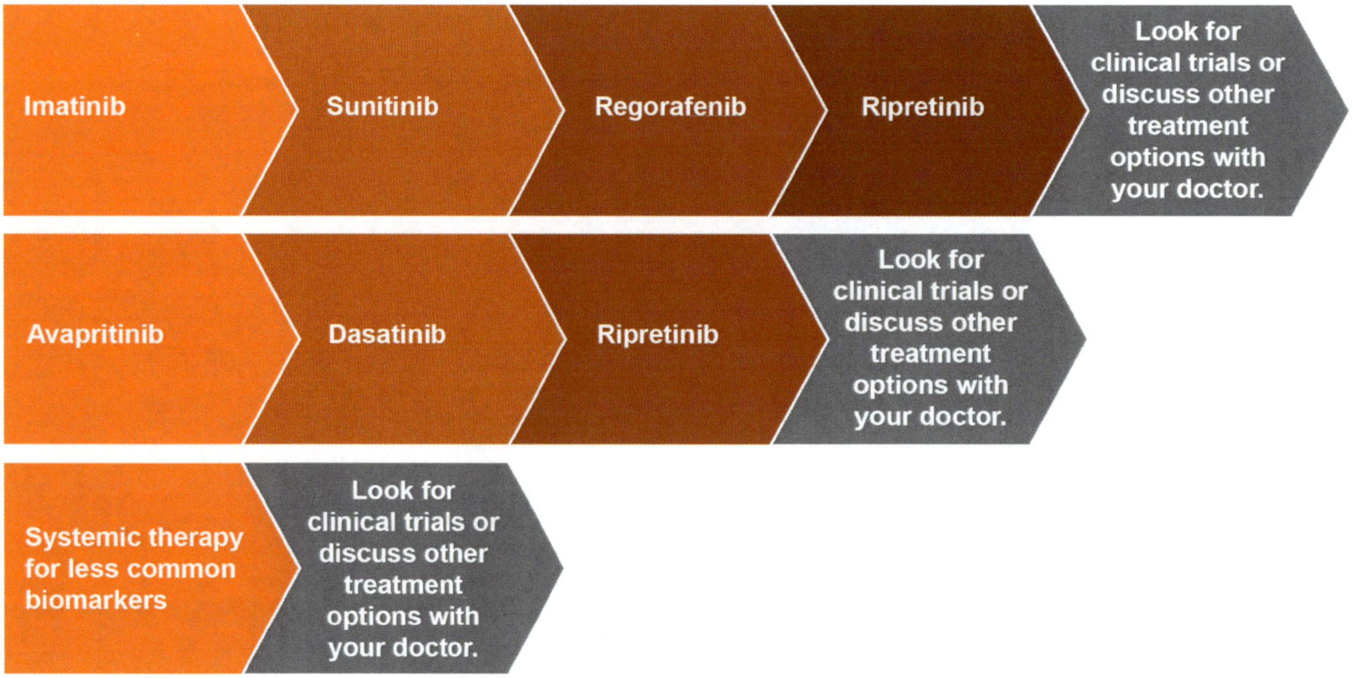

Local treatments

Ablation destroys small tumors. A special needle called a probe is placed into or next to the tumor, often with the help of an imaging test. The use of extreme cold (cryoablation) or extreme heat (e.g., microwave or radiofrequency ablation) to kill cancer cells is known as thermal ablation. Non-thermal types of ablation include irreversible electroporation (IRE), also known as "NanoKnife."

Embolization treats tumors by cutting off their blood supply. A catheter is inserted into an artery and guided to the tumor. Once in place, beads are inserted to block the blood flow. In **chemoembolization**, the beads are coated with chemotherapy. **Radioembolization** uses small radioactive beads.

open trials for which you may be eligible. See the next page for more information.

Best supportive care is always an option for progressive GIST. It is used alone or with other treatments to improve quality of life. This care might include reintroducing TKI therapy to help manage symptoms.

Clinical trials

A clinical trial is a type of medical research study. After being developed and tested in a laboratory, potential new ways of fighting cancer need to be studied in people. If found to be safe and effective in a clinical trial, a drug, device, or treatment approach may be approved by the U.S. Food and Drug Administration (FDA).

Everyone with cancer should carefully consider all of the treatment options available for their cancer type, including standard treatments and clinical trials. Talk to your doctor about whether a clinical trial may make sense for you.

Phases

Most cancer clinical trials focus on treatment. Treatment trials are done in phases.

- **Phase 1** trials study the dose, safety, and side effects of an investigational drug or treatment approach. They also look for early signs that the drug or approach is helpful.
- **Phase 2** trials study how well the drug or approach works against a specific type of cancer.
- **Phase 3** trials test the drug or approach against a standard treatment. If the results are good, it may be approved by the FDA.
- **Phase 4** trials study the long-term safety and benefit of an FDA-approved treatment.

Who can enroll?

Every clinical trial has rules for joining, called eligibility criteria. The rules may be about age, cancer type and stage, treatment history, or general health. These requirements ensure that participants are alike in specific ways and that the trial is as safe as possible for the participants.

Informed consent

Clinical trials are managed by a group of experts called a research team. The research team will review the study with you in detail, including its purpose and the risks and benefits of joining. All of this information is also provided in an informed consent form. Read the form carefully and ask questions before signing it. Take time to discuss it with family, friends, or others you trust. Keep in mind that you can leave and seek treatment outside of the clinical trial at any time.

Start the conversation

Don't wait for your doctor to bring up clinical trials. Start the conversation and learn about all of your treatment options. If you find a study you may be eligible for, ask your treatment team if you meet the requirements. If you have already started standard treatment, you may not be eligible for certain clinical trials. Try not to be discouraged if you cannot join. New clinical trials are always becoming available.

Frequently asked questions

There are many myths and misconceptions surrounding clinical trials. The possible benefits and risks are not well understood by many with cancer.

Will I get a placebo?

Placebos (inactive versions of real medicines) are almost never used alone in cancer clinical trials. It is common to receive either a placebo with a standard treatment or a new drug with a standard treatment. You will be informed, verbally and in writing, if a placebo is part of a clinical trial before you enroll.

Are clinical trials free?

There is no fee to enroll in a clinical trial. The study sponsor pays for research-related costs, including the study drug. You may, however, have costs indirectly related to the trial, such as the cost of transportation or child care due to extra appointments. During the trial, you will continue to receive standard cancer care.

Finding a clinical trial

In the United States

NCCN Cancer Centers
NCCN.org/cancercenters

The National Cancer Institute (NCI)
cancer.gov/about-cancer/treatment/clinical-trials/search

Worldwide

The U.S. National Library of Medicine (NLM)
clinicaltrials.gov

Need help finding a clinical trial?

NCI's Cancer Information Service (CIS)
1.800.4.CANCER (1.800.422.6237)
cancer.gov/contact

This care is billed to—and often covered by—insurance. You are responsible for copays and any costs for this care that are not covered by your insurance.

Key points

Treatment

- Surgery is recommended for GIST that are 2 cm or larger.
- No treatment is needed for very small, low-risk stomach GIST. You may have testing to monitor the size of the tumor. But surveillance instead of surgery has risks. Talk with your doctor about whether it is the best option for you.
- When possible, surgery is recommended for all other GIST. If surgery is too risky, you may have drug therapy first to shrink the tumor.
- If needed, the best drug treatment for you depends on the mutations and other features found during biomarker testing.
- Most GIST have either *KIT* or *PDGFRA* mutations. Imatinib is often the best choice for these tumors.
- Avapritinib is recommended for GIST with certain *PDGFRA* mutations that don't respond to imatinib, like D842V.
- Other options for drug therapy are available for GIST with the following biomarkers: *SDH*-deficiency, *NTRK* fusion-positive, and *BRAF* V600E mutation.

Surveillance after surgery

- After complete resection, a physical exam and CT scan are recommended every 3 to 6 months for 5 years after surgery.
- After 5 years, most people have imaging and a physical exam once per year.

Progression

- For GIST that progresses through all recommended drug therapies, consider enrolling in a clinical trial for treatment.
- Best supportive care is always an option for progressive GIST. It aims to improve quality of life.

3 Making treatment decisions

It's important to be comfortable with the cancer treatment you choose. This choice starts with having an open and honest conversation with your care team.

It's your choice

In shared decision-making, you and your doctors share information, discuss the options, and agree on a treatment plan. It starts with an open and honest conversation between you and your doctor.

Treatment decisions are very personal. What is important to you may not be important to someone else.

Some things that may play a role in your decision-making:

- What you want and how that might differ from what others want
- Your religious and spiritual beliefs
- Your feelings about certain treatments
- Your feelings about pain or side effects
- Cost of treatment, travel to treatment centers, and time away from school or work
- Quality of life and length of life
- How active you are and the activities that are important to you

Think about what you want from treatment. Discuss openly the risks and benefits of specific treatments and procedures. Weigh options and share concerns with your doctor.

If you take the time to build a relationship with your doctor, it will help you feel supported when considering options and making treatment decisions.

Second opinion

It is normal to want to start treatment as soon as possible. While cancer can't be ignored, there is time to have another doctor review your test results and suggest a treatment plan. This is called getting a second opinion, and it's a normal part of cancer care. Even doctors get second opinions!

Things you can do to prepare:

- Check with your insurance company about its rules on second opinions. There may be out-of-pocket costs to see doctors who are not part of your insurance plan.
- Make plans to have copies of all your records sent to the doctor you will see for your second opinion.

Support groups

Many people diagnosed with cancer find support groups to be helpful. Support groups often include people at different stages of treatment. Some people may be newly diagnosed, while others may be finished with treatment. If your hospital or community doesn't have support groups for people with cancer, check out the websites listed in this book.

Questions to ask

Possible questions to ask your doctors are listed on the following pages. Feel free to use these questions or come up with your own. Be clear about your goals for treatment and find out what to expect from treatment.

Questions about cancer testing

1. What tests will I have?
2. Do the tests have any risks?
3. Will my insurance pay for all of the tests you are recommending?
4. Do I need to do anything to prepare for testing?
5. Should I bring someone with me to the appointments?
6. Where do I go for testing, and how long will it take?
7. If any of the tests will hurt, what will you do to make me comfortable?
8. How soon will I know the results and who will explain them to me?
9. How can I get a copy of the pathology report and other test results?
10. Is there an online portal with my test results?

Questions about treatment options

1. What are my treatment options? What will happen if I do nothing?
2. Should I consider a clinical trial?
3. What is my prognosis?
4. Are you suggesting options other than what NCCN recommends? If yes, why?
5. How do my age, sex, overall health, and other factors affect my options?
6. What if I am pregnant, or planning to become pregnant?
7. Does any option offer a cure or long-term cancer control?
8. What are the side effects of the treatments?
9. How do I get a second opinion?
10. How long do I have to decide about treatment, and is there someone who can help me decide?

Questions about what to expect

1. Does this hospital or cancer center offer the best treatment for me?
2. Do I have a choice of when to begin treatment?
3. How long will treatment last?
4. Will my insurance cover the treatment you're recommending?
5. Are there any programs to help pay for treatment?
6. What supportive care and services are available to me?
7. Who should I contact with questions or concerns if the office is closed?
8. How will you know if treatment is working?
9. What are the chances of the cancer worsening or returning?
10. What follow-up care is needed after treatment?
11. Will I be able to continue working during treatment?

Questions about side effects

1. What are the possible complications and side effects of treatment?
2. Does the cancer itself cause any side effects?
3. Which side effects are most common and how long do they usually last?
4. Which side effects are serious or life-threatening?
5. Are there any long-term or permanent side effects?
6. What symptoms should I report right away, and who do I contact?
7. What can I do to prevent or relieve the side effects of treatment?
8. Do any medications worsen side effects?
9. Do any side effects lessen or worsen in severity over time?
10. Will you stop or change treatment if there are serious side effects?

Questions about clinical trials

1. Do you recommend that I consider a clinical trial for treatment?
2. How do I find a clinical trial?
3. What are the treatments used in the clinical trial?
4. Has the treatment been used for other types of cancer?
5. What are the risks and benefits of this treatment?
6. What side effects should I expect and how will they be managed?
7. How long will I be in the clinical trial?
8. Will I be able to get other treatment if this doesn't work?
9. How will you know if the treatment is working?
10. Will the clinical trial cost me anything?

Resources

Clear Cell Sarcoma Foundation
Clearcellsarcoma.org

Leiomyosarcoma Support & Direct Research Foundation
lmsdr.org

MSI Insiders
msiinsiders.org

National LeioMyoSarcoma Foundation
nlmsf.org

Northwest Sarcoma Foundation
nwsarcoma.org

Osteosarcoma Institute
osinst.org

Sarcoma Coalition
sarcomacoalition.us

Sarcoma Foundation of America
curesarcoma.org

The Life Raft Group
liferaftgroup.org

The Paula Takacs Foundation
paulatakacsfoundation.org

Triage Cancer
Triagecancer.org

Let us know what you think!

Please take a moment to complete an online survey about the NCCN Guidelines for Patients.

NCCN.org/patients/response

Words to know

ablation
A treatment that destroys very small tumors with heat, cold, lasers, or chemicals. Also called ablative therapy.

biomarker
A feature of a tumor or cancer that is used to guide treatment, often with systemic therapy. Tumor gene mutations often serve as biomarkers. Proteins made in response to the cancer can also be biomarkers.

***BRAF* V600E mutations**
A rare gene mutation found in GIST. A biomarker used to guide treatment with drug therapy.

cancer stage
A rating of the extent of cancer in the body.

chemoembolization
A cancer treatment with chemotherapy-coated beads that block blood supply to tumors.

cryoablation
Use of a special probe that destroys tumors by freezing them. A type of ablative therapy. Also called cryotherapy.

embolization
A treatment that cuts off blood supply to tumors with beads inserted into an artery.

endoscopic ultrasound-guided fine-needle aspiration biopsy (EUS-FNAB)
A procedure that removes fluid with a needle on an imaging device guided through a natural opening.

***KIT* mutation**
The most common gene mutation found in GIST. A biomarker used to guide treatment with drug therapy.

next-generation sequencing (NGS)
A method of biomarker testing that looks for a large group (panel) of mutations and other biomarkers at one time.

***NTRK* fusion**
A rare biomarker found in GIST.

***PDGFRA* mutation**
The second most common gene mutation found in GIST. A biomarker used to guide treatment with drug therapy.

radiofrequency ablation
A treatment that destroys cancer cells by heating them with high-energy radio waves.

sarcoma
A cancer of bone or soft tissue cells.

***SDH* deficiency**
A gene mutation often found in children and young adults with GIST. A biomarker used to guide treatment with drug therapy.

tyrosine kinase inhibitor (TKI)
The type of drug most commonly used treat GIST.

NCCN Contributors

This patient guide is based on the NCCN Clinical Practice Guidelines in Oncology (NCCN Guidelines®) for Gastrointestinal Stromal Tumors, Version 1.2023. It was adapted, reviewed, and published with help from the following people:

Dorothy A. Shead, MS
Senior Director
Patient Information Operations

Erin Vidic, MA
Senior Medical Writer, Patient Information

Laura Phillips
Graphic Design Specialist

The NCCN Guidelines® for Gastrointestinal Stromal Tumors, Version 1.2023 was developed by the following NCCN Panel Members:

Margaret von Mehren, MD/Chair
Fox Chase Cancer Center

John M. Kane, III, MD/Vice-Chair
Roswell Park Comprehensive Cancer Center

Samantha A. Armstrong, MD
Indiana University Melvin and Bren Simon Comprehensive Cancer Center

Andrew J. Bishop, MD
The University of Texas MD Anderson Cancer Center

Marilyn M. Bui, MD, PhD
Moffitt Cancer Center

Janai Carr-Ascher, MD, PhD
UC Davis Comprehensive Cancer Center

*Edwin Choy, MD, PhD
Massachusetts General Hospital Cancer Center

*Mary Connelly, LSW
The Ohio State University Comprehensive Cancer Center - James Cancer Hospital and Solove Research Institute

Sarah Dry, MD
UCLA Jonsson Comprehensive Cancer Center

Vanessa Eulo, MD
O'Neal Comprehensive Cancer Center at UAB

*Kristen N. Ganjoo, MD
Stanford Cancer Institute

Ricardo J. Gonzalez, MD
Moffitt Cancer Center

Ashley Holder, MD
O'Neal Comprehensive Cancer Center at UAB

Jade Homsi, MD
UT Southwestern Simmons Comprehensive Cancer Center

Vicki Keedy, MD, MSCI
Vanderbilt-Ingram Cancer Center

Ciara M. Kelly, MD
Memorial Sloan Kettering Cancer Center

Edward Kim, MD
Fred Hutchinson Cancer Center

David Liebner, MD
The Ohio State University Comprehensive Cancer Center - James Cancer Hospital and Solove Research Institute

Martin McCarter, MD
University of Colorado Cancer Center

Sean V. McGarry, MD
Fred & Pamela Buffett Cancer Center

Nathan W. Mesko, MD
Case Comprehensive Cancer Center/ University Hospitals Seidman Cancer Center and Cleveland Clinic Taussig Cancer Institute

Christian Meyer, MD, PhD
The Sidney Kimmel Comprehensive Cancer Center at Johns Hopkins

Alberto S. Pappo, MD
St. Jude Children's Research Hospital/The University of Tennessee Health Science Center

Ivy A. Petersen, MD
Mayo Clinic Comprehensive Cancer Center

Seth M. Pollack, MD
Robert H. Lurie Comprehensive Cancer Center of Northwestern University

Matthew Poppe, MD
Huntsman Cancer Institute at the University of Utah

*Richard F. Riedel, MD
Duke Cancer Institute

Scott Schuetze, MD, PhD
University of Michigan Rogel Cancer Center

Jacob Shabason, MD
Abramson Cancer Center at the University of Pennsylvania

*Jason K. Sicklick, MD
UC San Diego Moores Cancer Center

Lindsay Stratchko, DO
University of Wisconsin Carbone Cancer Center

William Tseng, MD
City of Hope National Medical Center

Brian A. Van Tine, MD, PhD
Siteman Cancer Center at Barnes-Jewish Hospital and Washington University School of Medicine

Melissa Zimel, MD
UCSF Helen Diller Family Comprehensive Cancer Center

NCCN

Lisa E. Hang, PhD
Oncology Scientist/Medical Writer

Mary Anne Bergman
Guidelines Coordinator

* Reviewed this patient guide. For disclosures, visit NCCN.org/disclosures.

NCCN Cancer Centers

Abramson Cancer Center
at the University of Pennsylvania
Philadelphia, Pennsylvania
800.789.7366 • pennmedicine.org/cancer

Case Comprehensive Cancer Center/
University Hospitals Seidman Cancer Center
and Cleveland Clinic Taussig Cancer Institute
Cleveland, Ohio
UH Seidman Cancer Center
800.641.2422 • uhhospitals.org/services/cancer-services
CC Taussig Cancer Institute
866.223.8100 • my.clevelandclinic.org/departments/cancer
Case CCC
216.844.8797 • case.edu/cancer

City of Hope National Medical Center
Duarte, California
800.826.4673 • cityofhope.org

Dana-Farber/Brigham and Women's Cancer Center |
Massachusetts General Hospital Cancer Center
Boston, Massachusetts
617.732.5500 • youhaveus.org
617.726.5130 • massgeneral.org/cancer-center

Duke Cancer Institute
Durham, North Carolina
888.275.3853 • dukecancerinstitute.org

Fox Chase Cancer Center
Philadelphia, Pennsylvania
888.369.2427 • foxchase.org

Fred & Pamela Buffett Cancer Center
Omaha, Nebraska
402.559.5600 • unmc.edu/cancercenter

Fred Hutchinson Cancer Center
Seattle, Washington
206.667.5000 • fredhutch.org

Huntsman Cancer Institute at the University of Utah
Salt Lake City, Utah
800.824.2073 • huntsmancancer.org

Indiana University Melvin and Bren Simon
Comprehensive Cancer Center
Indianapolis, Indiana
888.600.4822 • www.cancer.iu.edu

Mayo Clinic Comprehensive Cancer Center
Phoenix/Scottsdale, Arizona
Jacksonville, Florida
Rochester, Minnesota
480.301.8000 • Arizona
904.953.0853 • Florida
507.538.3270 • Minnesota
mayoclinic.org/cancercenter

Memorial Sloan Kettering Cancer Center
New York, New York
800.525.2225 • mskcc.org

Moffitt Cancer Center
Tampa, Florida
888.663.3488 • moffitt.org

O'Neal Comprehensive Cancer Center at UAB
Birmingham, Alabama
800.822.0933 • uab.edu/onealcancercenter

Robert H. Lurie Comprehensive Cancer
Center of Northwestern University
Chicago, Illinois
866.587.4322 • cancer.northwestern.edu

Roswell Park Comprehensive Cancer Center
Buffalo, New York
877.275.7724 • roswellpark.org

Siteman Cancer Center at Barnes-Jewish Hospital
and Washington University School of Medicine
St. Louis, Missouri
800.600.3606 • siteman.wustl.edu

St. Jude Children's Research Hospital/
The University of Tennessee Health Science Center
Memphis, Tennessee
866.278.5833 • stjude.org
901.448.5500 • uthsc.edu

Stanford Cancer Institute
Stanford, California
877.668.7535 • cancer.stanford.edu

The Ohio State University Comprehensive
Cancer Center - James Cancer Hospital
and Solove Research Institute
Columbus, Ohio
800.293.5066 • cancer.osu.edu

The Sidney Kimmel Comprehensive
Cancer Center at Johns Hopkins
Baltimore, Maryland
410.955.8964
www.hopkinskimmelcancercenter.org

The UChicago Medicine Comprehensive Cancer Center
Chicago, Illinois
773.702.1000 • uchicagomedicine.org/cancer

The University of Texas MD Anderson Cancer Center
Houston, Texas
844.269.5922 • mdanderson.org

UC Davis Comprehensive Cancer Center
Sacramento, California
916.734.5959 • 800.770.9261
health.ucdavis.edu/cancer

UC San Diego Moores Cancer Center
La Jolla, California
858.822.6100 • cancer.ucsd.edu

UCLA Jonsson Comprehensive Cancer Center
Los Angeles, California
310.825.5268 • cancer.ucla.edu

UCSF Helen Diller Family
Comprehensive Cancer Center
San Francisco, California
800.689.8273 • cancer.ucsf.edu

University of Colorado Cancer Center
Aurora, Colorado
720.848.0300 • coloradocancercenter.org

University of Michigan Rogel Cancer Center
Ann Arbor, Michigan
800.865.1125 • rogelcancercenter.org

University of Wisconsin Carbone Cancer Center
Madison, Wisconsin
608.265.1700 • uwhealth.org/cancer

UT Southwestern Simmons
Comprehensive Cancer Center
Dallas, Texas
214.648.3111 • utsouthwestern.edu/simmons

Vanderbilt-Ingram Cancer Center
Nashville, Tennessee
877.936.8422 • vicc.org

Yale Cancer Center/Smilow Cancer Hospital
New Haven, Connecticut
855.4.SMILOW • yalecancercenter.org

Notes

Index

Made in the USA
Coppell, TX
30 September 2026

91414136R00021